GRATITU
and
MINDFULNESS
JOURNAL

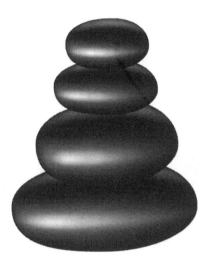

This Journal Belongs to:

_____

ISBN: 978-1-952358-17-3

Limits of Liability and Disclaimer of Warranty
The author and publisher shall not be liable for your misuse
of this material. This book is strictly for informational
and educational purposes.

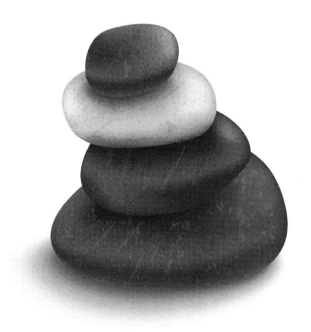

To the mind that is still,
the whole universe surrenders.
— Lao Tzu

He who would be serene and pure needs but one thing,
detachment. — Meister Eckhart

Day: _____   Date: __/__/____

1. Today's message to myself:

_____

2. Someone I could surprise with a note, gift or sign of appreciation and why:

_____

3. Today I am grateful for:

_____

_____

_____

_____

Day: _____   Date: __/__/____

1. Today's message to myself:

_____

2. Someone I could surprise with a note, gift or sign of appreciation and why:

_____

3. Today I am grateful for:

_____

_____

_____

_____

Day: _____   Date: __/__/____

1. Today's message to myself:

_____

2. Someone I could surprise with a note, gift or sign of appreciation and why:

_____

3. Today I am grateful for:

_____

_____

_____

_____

To forget oneself is to be happy.
— Robert Louis Stevenson

Day: _____   Date: __/__/___

1. Today's message to myself:

_____

2. Someone I could surprise with a note, gift or sign of appreciation and why:

_____

3. Today I am grateful for:

_____

_____

_____

_____

Day: _____   Date: __/__/___

1. Today's message to myself:

_____

2. Someone I could surprise with a note, gift or sign of appreciation and why:

_____

3. Today I am grateful for:

_____

_____

_____

_____

Day: _____   Date: __/__/___

1. Today's message to myself:

_____

2. Someone I could surprise with a note, gift or sign of appreciation and why:

_____

3. Today I am grateful for:

_____

_____

_____

_____

The eye sees what it brings the power to see.
— Thomas Carlyle

Day: _____   Date: __/__/___

1. Today's message to myself:

_____

2. Someone I could surprise with a note, gift or sign of appreciation and why:

_____

3. Today I am grateful for:

_____

_____

_____

_____

Day: _____   Date: __/__/___

1. Today's message to myself:

_____

2. Someone I could surprise with a note, gift or sign of appreciation and why:

_____

3. Today I am grateful for:

_____

_____

_____

_____

Day: _____   Date: __/__/___

1. Today's message to myself:

_____

2. Someone I could surprise with a note, gift or sign of appreciation and why:

_____

3. Today I am grateful for:

_____

_____

_____

_____

There is no harm in repeating a good thing.
— Plato

Day: _____   Date: __/__/___

1. Today's message to myself:
_____

2. Someone I could surprise with a note, gift or sign of appreciation and why:
_____

3. Today I am grateful for:
_____
_____
_____
_____

Day: _____   Date: __/__/___

1. Today's message to myself:
_____

2. Someone I could surprise with a note, gift or sign of appreciation and why:
_____

3. Today I am grateful for:
_____
_____
_____
_____

Day: _____   Date: __/__/___

1. Today's message to myself:
_____

2. Someone I could surprise with a note, gift or sign of appreciation and why:
_____

3. Today I am grateful for:
_____
_____
_____
_____

The best thing one can do when it's raining is to let it rain.
— Henry Wadsworth Longfellow

Day: _____   Date: __/__/___

1. Today's message to myself:
_____

2. Someone I could surprise with a note, gift or sign of appreciation and why:
_____

3. Today I am grateful for:
_____
_____
_____
_____

Day: _____   Date: __/__/___

1. Today's message to myself:
_____

2. Someone I could surprise with a note, gift or sign of appreciation and why:
_____

3. Today I am grateful for:
_____
_____
_____
_____

Day: _____   Date: __/__/___

1. Today's message to myself:
_____

2. Someone I could surprise with a note, gift or sign of appreciation and why:
_____

3. Today I am grateful for:
_____
_____
_____
_____

Find ecstasy in life; the mere sense of living is joy enough.
— Emily Dickinson

Day: _____   Date: __/__/____

1. Today's message to myself:
_____

2. Someone I could surprise with a note, gift or sign of appreciation and why:
_____

3. Today I am grateful for:
_____
_____
_____
_____

Day: _____   Date: __/__/____

1. Today's message to myself:
_____

2. Someone I could surprise with a note, gift or sign of appreciation and why:
_____

3. Today I am grateful for:
_____
_____
_____
_____

Day: _____   Date: __/__/____

1. Today's message to myself:
_____

2. Someone I could surprise with a note, gift or sign of appreciation and why:
_____

3. Today I am grateful for:
_____
_____
_____
_____

He who cannot give anything away cannot feel anything either.
— Friedrich Nietzsche

Day: _____   Date: _/_/___

1. Today's message to myself:

_____

2. Someone I could surprise with a note, gift or sign of appreciation and why:

_____

3. Today I am grateful for:

_____

_____

_____

_____

Day: _____   Date: _/_/___

1. Today's message to myself:

_____

2. Someone I could surprise with a note, gift or sign of appreciation and why:

_____

3. Today I am grateful for:

_____

_____

_____

_____

Day: _____   Date: _/_/___

1. Today's message to myself:

_____

2. Someone I could surprise with a note, gift or sign of appreciation and why:

_____

3. Today I am grateful for:

_____

_____

_____

How glorious a greeting the sun gives the mountains!
— John Muir

Day: _____   Date: __/__/___

1. Today's message to myself:

_____

2. Someone I could surprise with a note, gift or sign of appreciation and why:

_____

3. Today I am grateful for:

_____

_____

_____

_____

Day: _____   Date: __/__/___

1. Today's message to myself:

_____

2. Someone I could surprise with a note, gift or sign of appreciation and why:

_____

3. Today I am grateful for:

_____

_____

_____

_____

Day: _____   Date: __/__/___

1. Today's message to myself:

_____

2. Someone I could surprise with a note, gift or sign of appreciation and why:

_____

3. Today I am grateful for:

_____

_____

_____

_____

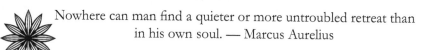

Nowhere can man find a quieter or more untroubled retreat than in his own soul. — Marcus Aurelius

Day: _____   Date: _/_/___

1. Today's message to myself:

_____

2. Someone I could surprise with a note, gift or sign of appreciation and why:

_____

3. Today I am grateful for:

_____

_____

_____

_____

Day: _____   Date: _/_/___

1. Today's message to myself:

_____

2. Someone I could surprise with a note, gift or sign of appreciation and why:

_____

3. Today I am grateful for:

_____

_____

_____

_____

Day: _____   Date: _/_/___

1. Today's message to myself:

_____

2. Someone I could surprise with a note, gift or sign of appreciation and why:

_____

3. Today I am grateful for:

_____

_____

_____

_____

You cannot do a kindness too soon, for you never know how soon it will be too late. — Ralph Waldo Emerson

Day: _____   Date: __/__/___

1. Today's message to myself:
_____

2. Someone I could surprise with a note, gift or sign of appreciation and why:
_____

3. Today I am grateful for:
_____
_____
_____
_____

Day: _____   Date: __/__/___

1. Today's message to myself:
_____

2. Someone I could surprise with a note, gift or sign of appreciation and why:
_____

3. Today I am grateful for:
_____
_____
_____
_____

Day: _____   Date: __/__/___

1. Today's message to myself:
_____

2. Someone I could surprise with a note, gift or sign of appreciation and why:
_____

3. Today I am grateful for:
_____
_____
_____
_____

Imagination is the eye of the soul.
— Joseph Joubert

Day: _____   Date: __/__/___

1. Today's message to myself:
_____

2. Someone I could surprise with a note, gift or sign of appreciation and why:
_____

3. Today I am grateful for:
_____
_____
_____
_____

Day: _____   Date: __/__/___

1. Today's message to myself:
_____

2. Someone I could surprise with a note, gift or sign of appreciation and why:
_____

3. Today I am grateful for:
_____
_____
_____
_____

Day: _____   Date: __/__/___

1. Today's message to myself:
_____

2. Someone I could surprise with a note, gift or sign of appreciation and why:
_____

3. Today I am grateful for:
_____
_____
_____
_____

Be as you wish to seem.
— Socrates

Day: _____   Date: __/__/____

1. Today's message to myself:

_____

2. Someone I could surprise with a note, gift or sign of appreciation and why:

_____

3. Today I am grateful for:

_____

_____

_____

_____

Day: _____   Date: __/__/____

1. Today's message to myself:

_____

2. Someone I could surprise with a note, gift or sign of appreciation and why:

_____

3. Today I am grateful for:

_____

_____

_____

_____

Day: _____   Date: __/__/____

1. Today's message to myself:

_____

2. Someone I could surprise with a note, gift or sign of appreciation and why:

_____

3. Today I am grateful for:

_____

_____

_____

_____

Life can only be understood backwards; but it must be
lived forwards. — Soren Kierkegaard

Day: _____   Date: __/__/___

1. Today's message to myself:
_____

2. Someone I could surprise with a note, gift or sign of appreciation and why:
_____

3. Today I am grateful for:
_____
_____
_____
_____

Day: _____   Date: __/__/___

1. Today's message to myself:
_____

2. Someone I could surprise with a note, gift or sign of appreciation and why:
_____

3. Today I am grateful for:
_____
_____
_____
_____

Day: _____   Date: __/__/___

1. Today's message to myself:
_____

2. Someone I could surprise with a note, gift or sign of appreciation and why:
_____

3. Today I am grateful for:
_____
_____
_____

A Moment of Mindfulness

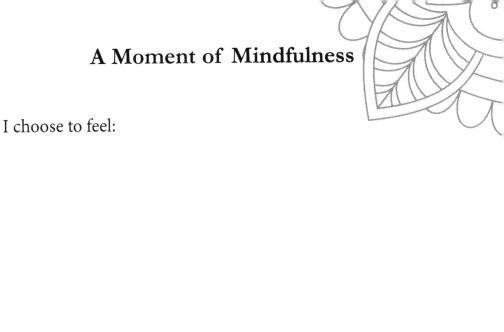

I choose to feel:

My focus:

I feel inspired by:

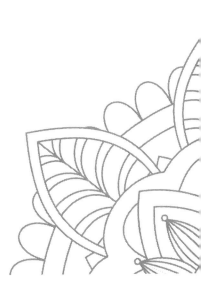

Act as if what you do makes a difference. It does.
— William James

Day: _____   Date: __/__/____

1. Today's message to myself:
_____

2. Someone I could surprise with a note, gift or sign of appreciation and why:
_____

3. Today I am grateful for:
_____
_____
_____
_____

Day: _____   Date: __/__/____

1. Today's message to myself:
_____

2. Someone I could surprise with a note, gift or sign of appreciation and why:
_____

3. Today I am grateful for:
_____
_____
_____
_____

Day: _____   Date: __/__/____

1. Today's message to myself:
_____

2. Someone I could surprise with a note, gift or sign of appreciation and why:
_____

3. Today I am grateful for:
_____
_____
_____

Day: _____   Date: __/__/____

1. Today's message to myself:

_____

2. Someone I could surprise with a note, gift or sign of appreciation and why:

_____

3. Today I am grateful for:

_____

_____

_____

_____

Day: _____   Date: __/__/____

1. Today's message to myself:

_____

2. Someone I could surprise with a note, gift or sign of appreciation and why:

_____

3. Today I am grateful for:

_____

_____

_____

_____

Day: _____   Date: __/__/____

1. Today's message to myself:

_____

2. Someone I could surprise with a note, gift or sign of appreciation and why:

_____

3. Today I am grateful for:

_____

_____

_____

_____

To love oneself is the beginning of a lifelong romance.
— Oscar Wilde

Day: _____   Date: _/_/____

1. Today's message to myself:

_____

2. Someone I could surprise with a note, gift or sign of appreciation and why:

_____

3. Today I am grateful for:

_____

_____

_____

_____

Day: _____   Date: _/_/____

1. Today's message to myself:

_____

2. Someone I could surprise with a note, gift or sign of appreciation and why:

_____

3. Today I am grateful for:

_____

_____

_____

_____

Day: _____   Date: _/_/____

1. Today's message to myself:

_____

2. Someone I could surprise with a note, gift or sign of appreciation and why:

_____

3. Today I am grateful for:

_____

_____

_____

_____

To be is to do.
— Immanuel Kant

Day: _____ Date: __/__/___

1. Today's message to myself:
_____

2. Someone I could surprise with a note, gift or sign of appreciation and why:
_____

3. Today I am grateful for:
_____
_____
_____
_____

Day: _____ Date: __/__/___

1. Today's message to myself:
_____

2. Someone I could surprise with a note, gift or sign of appreciation and why:
_____

3. Today I am grateful for:
_____
_____
_____
_____

Day: _____ Date: __/__/___

1. Today's message to myself:
_____

2. Someone I could surprise with a note, gift or sign of appreciation and why:
_____

3. Today I am grateful for:
_____
_____
_____
_____

We feel and know that we are eternal.
— Baruch Spinoza

Day: _____   Date: __/__/___

1. Today's message to myself:
_____

2. Someone I could surprise with a note, gift or sign of appreciation and why:
_____

3. Today I am grateful for:
_____
_____
_____

Day: _____   Date: __/__/___

1. Today's message to myself:
_____

2. Someone I could surprise with a note, gift or sign of appreciation and why:
_____

3. Today I am grateful for:
_____
_____
_____

Day: _____   Date: __/__/___

1. Today's message to myself:
_____

2. Someone I could surprise with a note, gift or sign of appreciation and why:
_____

3. Today I am grateful for:
_____
_____
_____

There are two ways of spreading light: to be the candle or the mirror
that reflects it. — Edith Wharton

Day: _____   Date: __/__/___

1. Today's message to myself:
_____

2. Someone I could surprise with a note, gift or sign of appreciation and why:
_____

3. Today I am grateful for:
_____

_____

_____

Day: _____   Date: __/__/___

1. Today's message to myself:
_____

2. Someone I could surprise with a note, gift or sign of appreciation and why:
_____

3. Today I am grateful for:
_____

_____

_____

Day: _____   Date: __/__/___

1. Today's message to myself:
_____

2. Someone I could surprise with a note, gift or sign of appreciation and why:
_____

3. Today I am grateful for:
_____

_____

_____

Things alter for the worse spontaneously, if they be not altered for the better designedly. — Francis Bacon

Day: _____   Date: __/__/____

1. Today's message to myself:
_____

2. Someone I could surprise with a note, gift or sign of appreciation and why:
_____

3. Today I am grateful for:
_____
_____
_____
_____

Day: _____   Date: __/__/____

1. Today's message to myself:
_____

2. Someone I could surprise with a note, gift or sign of appreciation and why:
_____

3. Today I am grateful for:
_____
_____
_____
_____

Day: _____   Date: __/__/____

1. Today's message to myself:
_____

2. Someone I could surprise with a note, gift or sign of appreciation and why:
_____

3. Today I am grateful for:
_____
_____
_____
_____

You and I do not see things as they are. We see things as we are.
— Henry Ward Beecher

Day: _____   Date: __/__/____

1. Today's message to myself:
_____

2. Someone I could surprise with a note, gift or sign of appreciation and why:
_____

3. Today I am grateful for:
_____
_____
_____
_____

Day: _____   Date: __/__/____

1. Today's message to myself:
_____

2. Someone I could surprise with a note, gift or sign of appreciation and why:
_____

3. Today I am grateful for:
_____
_____
_____
_____

Day: _____   Date: __/__/____

1. Today's message to myself:
_____

2. Someone I could surprise with a note, gift or sign of appreciation and why:
_____

3. Today I am grateful for:
_____
_____
_____
_____

It is never too late to be what you might have been.
— George Eliot

Day: _____   Date: __/__/____

1. Today's message to myself:

_____

2. Someone I could surprise with a note, gift or sign of appreciation and why:

_____

3. Today I am grateful for:

_____

_____

_____

_____

Day: _____   Date: __/__/____

1. Today's message to myself:

_____

2. Someone I could surprise with a note, gift or sign of appreciation and why:

_____

3. Today I am grateful for:

_____

_____

_____

_____

Day: _____   Date: __/__/____

1. Today's message to myself:

_____

2. Someone I could surprise with a note, gift or sign of appreciation and why:

_____

3. Today I am grateful for:

_____

_____

_____

The clearest way into the Universe is through a forest wilderness.
— John Muir

Day: _____   Date: __/__/___

1. Today's message to myself:

_____

2. Someone I could surprise with a note, gift or sign of appreciation and why:

_____

3. Today I am grateful for:

_____

_____

_____

_____

Day: _____   Date: __/__/___

1. Today's message to myself:

_____

2. Someone I could surprise with a note, gift or sign of appreciation and why:

_____

3. Today I am grateful for:

_____

_____

_____

_____

Day: _____   Date: __/__/___

1. Today's message to myself:

_____

2. Someone I could surprise with a note, gift or sign of appreciation and why:

_____

3. Today I am grateful for:

_____

_____

_____

_____

Rejoice in the things that are present; all else is beyond thee.
— Michel de Montaigne

Day: _____   Date: _/_/___

1. Today's message to myself:

_____

2. Someone I could surprise with a note, gift or sign of appreciation and why:

_____

3. Today I am grateful for:

_____
_____
_____
_____

Day: _____   Date: _/_/___

1. Today's message to myself:

_____

2. Someone I could surprise with a note, gift or sign of appreciation and why:

_____

3. Today I am grateful for:

_____
_____
_____
_____

Day: _____   Date: _/_/___

1. Today's message to myself:

_____

2. Someone I could surprise with a note, gift or sign of appreciation and why:

_____

3. Today I am grateful for:

_____
_____
_____
_____

Nothing great was ever achieved without enthusiasm.
— Ralph Waldo Emerson

Day: _____   Date: __/__/____

1. Today's message to myself:
_____

2. Someone I could surprise with a note, gift or sign of appreciation and why:
_____

3. Today I am grateful for:
_____
_____
_____
_____

Day: _____   Date: __/__/____

1. Today's message to myself:
_____

2. Someone I could surprise with a note, gift or sign of appreciation and why:
_____

3. Today I am grateful for:
_____
_____
_____
_____

Day: _____   Date: __/__/____

1. Today's message to myself:
_____

2. Someone I could surprise with a note, gift or sign of appreciation and why:
_____

3. Today I am grateful for:
_____
_____
_____

Life must be lived as play.
— Plato

Day: _____   Date: __/__/____

1. Today's message to myself:

_____

2. Someone I could surprise with a note, gift or sign of appreciation and why:

_____

3. Today I am grateful for:

_____

_____

_____

_____

Day: _____   Date: __/__/____

1. Today's message to myself:

_____

2. Someone I could surprise with a note, gift or sign of appreciation and why:

_____

3. Today I am grateful for:

_____

_____

_____

_____

Day: _____   Date: __/__/____

1. Today's message to myself:

_____

2. Someone I could surprise with a note, gift or sign of appreciation and why:

_____

3. Today I am grateful for:

_____

_____

_____

A Moment of Mindfulness

What are my thoughts?

What emotion do I attach to these thoughts?

Can I let it go ...

You can give without loving, but you can never love
without giving. — Robert Louis Stevenson

Day: _____   Date: __/__/____

1. Today's message to myself:

_____

2. Someone I could surprise with a note, gift or sign of appreciation and why:

_____

3. Today I am grateful for:

_____

_____

_____

_____

Day: _____   Date: __/__/____

1. Today's message to myself:

_____

2. Someone I could surprise with a note, gift or sign of appreciation and why:

_____

3. Today I am grateful for:

_____

_____

_____

_____

Day: _____   Date: __/__/____

1. Today's message to myself:

_____

2. Someone I could surprise with a note, gift or sign of appreciation and why:

_____

3. Today I am grateful for:

_____

_____

_____

They can conquer who believe they can.
— Virgil

Day: _____   Date: __/__/____

1. Today's message to myself:
_____

2. Someone I could surprise with a note, gift or sign of appreciation and why:
_____

3. Today I am grateful for:
_____
_____
_____
_____

Day: _____   Date: __/__/____

1. Today's message to myself:
_____

2. Someone I could surprise with a note, gift or sign of appreciation and why:
_____

3. Today I am grateful for:
_____
_____
_____
_____

Day: _____   Date: __/__/____

1. Today's message to myself:
_____

2. Someone I could surprise with a note, gift or sign of appreciation and why:
_____

3. Today I am grateful for:
_____
_____
_____
_____

A gentle word, a kind look, a good-natured smile can work wonders and accomplish miracles. — William Hazlitt

Day: _____   Date: __/__/____

1. Today's message to myself:

_____

2. Someone I could surprise with a note, gift or sign of appreciation and why:

_____

3. Today I am grateful for:

_____

_____

_____

_____

Day: _____   Date: __/__/____

1. Today's message to myself:

_____

2. Someone I could surprise with a note, gift or sign of appreciation and why:

_____

3. Today I am grateful for:

_____

_____

_____

_____

Day: _____   Date: __/__/____

1. Today's message to myself:

_____

2. Someone I could surprise with a note, gift or sign of appreciation and why:

_____

3. Today I am grateful for:

_____

_____

_____

> Wonder is the desire for knowledge.
> — Thomas Aquinas

Day: _____   Date: __/__/____

1. Today's message to myself:

_____

2. Someone I could surprise with a note, gift or sign of appreciation and why:

_____

3. Today I am grateful for:

_____

_____

_____

_____

Day: _____   Date: __/__/____

1. Today's message to myself:

_____

2. Someone I could surprise with a note, gift or sign of appreciation and why:

_____

3. Today I am grateful for:

_____

_____

_____

_____

Day: _____   Date: __/__/____

1. Today's message to myself:

_____

2. Someone I could surprise with a note, gift or sign of appreciation and why:

_____

3. Today I am grateful for:

_____

_____

_____

_____

Our happiness depends on wisdom all the way.
— Sophocles

Day: _____   Date: __/__/___

1. Today's message to myself:
_____

2. Someone I could surprise with a note, gift or sign of appreciation and why:
_____

3. Today I am grateful for:
_____
_____
_____
_____

Day: _____   Date: __/__/___

1. Today's message to myself:
_____

2. Someone I could surprise with a note, gift or sign of appreciation and why:
_____

3. Today I am grateful for:
_____
_____
_____
_____

Day: _____   Date: __/__/___

1. Today's message to myself:
_____

2. Someone I could surprise with a note, gift or sign of appreciation and why:
_____

3. Today I am grateful for:
_____
_____
_____

If it were not for hopes, the heart would break.
— Thomas Fuller

Day: _____   Date: __/__/____

1. Today's message to myself:
_____

2. Someone I could surprise with a note, gift or sign of appreciation and why:
_____

3. Today I am grateful for:
_____
_____
_____
_____

Day: _____   Date: __/__/____

1. Today's message to myself:
_____

2. Someone I could surprise with a note, gift or sign of appreciation and why:
_____

3. Today I am grateful for:
_____
_____
_____
_____

Day: _____   Date: __/__/____

1. Today's message to myself:
_____

2. Someone I could surprise with a note, gift or sign of appreciation and why:
_____

3. Today I am grateful for:
_____
_____
_____

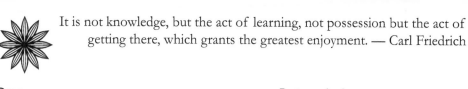

It is not knowledge, but the act of learning, not possession but the act of getting there, which grants the greatest enjoyment. — Carl Friedrich

Day: _____   Date: __/__/___

1. Today's message to myself:

_____

2. Someone I could surprise with a note, gift or sign of appreciation and why:

_____

3. Today I am grateful for:

_____

_____

_____

_____

Day: _____   Date: __/__/___

1. Today's message to myself:

_____

2. Someone I could surprise with a note, gift or sign of appreciation and why:

_____

3. Today I am grateful for:

_____

_____

_____

_____

Day: _____   Date: __/__/___

1. Today's message to myself:

_____

2. Someone I could surprise with a note, gift or sign of appreciation and why:

_____

3. Today I am grateful for:

_____

_____

_____

_____

I hear and I forget. I see and I remember. I do and I understand.
— Confucius

Day: _____   Date: __/__/___

1. Today's message to myself:

_____

2. Someone I could surprise with a note, gift or sign of appreciation and why:

_____

3. Today I am grateful for:

_____
_____
_____
_____

Day: _____   Date: __/__/___

1. Today's message to myself:

_____

2. Someone I could surprise with a note, gift or sign of appreciation and why:

_____

3. Today I am grateful for:

_____
_____
_____
_____

Day: _____   Date: __/__/___

1. Today's message to myself:

_____

2. Someone I could surprise with a note, gift or sign of appreciation and why:

_____

3. Today I am grateful for:

_____
_____
_____
_____

Happiness depends upon ourselves.
— Aristotle

Day: _____   Date: __/__/____

1. Today's message to myself:

_____

2. Someone I could surprise with a note, gift or sign of appreciation and why:

_____

3. Today I am grateful for:

_____

_____

_____

_____

Day: _____   Date: __/__/____

1. Today's message to myself:

_____

2. Someone I could surprise with a note, gift or sign of appreciation and why:

_____

3. Today I am grateful for:

_____

_____

_____

_____

Day: _____   Date: __/__/____

1. Today's message to myself:

_____

2. Someone I could surprise with a note, gift or sign of appreciation and why:

_____

3. Today I am grateful for:

_____

_____

_____

Excessive fear is always powerless.
— Aeschylus

Day: _____   Date: __/__/___

1. Today's message to myself:
_____

2. Someone I could surprise with a note, gift or sign of appreciation and why:
_____

3. Today I am grateful for:
_____
_____
_____
_____

Day: _____   Date: __/__/___

1. Today's message to myself:
_____

2. Someone I could surprise with a note, gift or sign of appreciation and why:
_____

3. Today I am grateful for:
_____
_____
_____
_____

Day: _____   Date: __/__/___

1. Today's message to myself:
_____

2. Someone I could surprise with a note, gift or sign of appreciation and why:
_____

3. Today I am grateful for:
_____
_____
_____

We would often be sorry if our wishes were gratified.
— Aesop

Day: _____   Date: _/_/___

1. Today's message to myself:

_____

2. Someone I could surprise with a note, gift or sign of appreciation and why:

_____

3. Today I am grateful for:

_____

_____

_____

_____

Day: _____   Date: _/_/___

1. Today's message to myself:

_____

2. Someone I could surprise with a note, gift or sign of appreciation and why:

_____

3. Today I am grateful for:

_____

_____

_____

_____

Day: _____   Date: _/_/___

1. Today's message to myself:

_____

2. Someone I could surprise with a note, gift or sign of appreciation and why:

_____

3. Today I am grateful for:

_____

_____

_____

Day: _____   Date: __/__/____

1. Today's message to myself:

_____

2. Someone I could surprise with a note, gift or sign of appreciation and why:

_____

3. Today I am grateful for:

_____

_____

_____

_____

Day: _____   Date: __/__/____

1. Today's message to myself:

_____

2. Someone I could surprise with a note, gift or sign of appreciation and why:

_____

3. Today I am grateful for:

_____

_____

_____

_____

Day: _____   Date: __/__/____

1. Today's message to myself:

_____

2. Someone I could surprise with a note, gift or sign of appreciation and why:

_____

3. Today I am grateful for:

_____

_____

_____

_____

Happiness resides not in possessions, and not in gold,
happiness dwells in the soul. — Democritus

Day: _____   Date: __/__/___

1. Today's message to myself:
_____

2. Someone I could surprise with a note, gift or sign of appreciation and why:
_____

3. Today I am grateful for:
_____
_____
_____
_____

Day: _____   Date: __/__/___

1. Today's message to myself:
_____

2. Someone I could surprise with a note, gift or sign of appreciation and why:
_____

3. Today I am grateful for:
_____
_____
_____
_____

Day: _____   Date: __/__/___

1. Today's message to myself:
_____

2. Someone I could surprise with a note, gift or sign of appreciation and why:
_____

3. Today I am grateful for:
_____
_____
_____
_____

A Moment of Mindfulness

I choose to allow:

I choose to receive:

I am:

It is during our darkest moments that we must focus to
see the light. — Aristotle

Day: _____   Date: __/__/____

1. Today's message to myself:

_____

2. Someone I could surprise with a note, gift or sign of appreciation and why:

_____

3. Today I am grateful for:

_____

_____

_____

_____

Day: _____   Date: __/__/____

1. Today's message to myself:

_____

2. Someone I could surprise with a note, gift or sign of appreciation and why:

_____

3. Today I am grateful for:

_____

_____

_____

_____

Day: _____   Date: __/__/____

1. Today's message to myself:

_____

2. Someone I could surprise with a note, gift or sign of appreciation and why:

_____

3. Today I am grateful for:

_____

_____

_____

_____

No great thing is created suddenly.
— Epictetus

Day: _____   Date: __/__/____

1. Today's message to myself:
_____

2. Someone I could surprise with a note, gift or sign of appreciation and why:
_____

3. Today I am grateful for:
_____
_____
_____
_____

Day: _____   Date: __/__/____

1. Today's message to myself:
_____

2. Someone I could surprise with a note, gift or sign of appreciation and why:
_____

3. Today I am grateful for:
_____
_____
_____
_____

Day: _____   Date: __/__/____

1. Today's message to myself:
_____

2. Someone I could surprise with a note, gift or sign of appreciation and why:
_____

3. Today I am grateful for:
_____
_____
_____

The dawn is not distant, nor is the night starless; love is eternal.
— Henry Wadsworth Longfellow

Day: _____   Date: __/__/____

1. Today's message to myself:
_____

2. Someone I could surprise with a note, gift or sign of appreciation and why:
_____

3. Today I am grateful for:
_____
_____
_____
_____

Day: _____   Date: __/__/____

1. Today's message to myself:
_____

2. Someone I could surprise with a note, gift or sign of appreciation and why:
_____

3. Today I am grateful for:
_____
_____
_____
_____

Day: _____   Date: __/__/____

1. Today's message to myself:
_____

2. Someone I could surprise with a note, gift or sign of appreciation and why:
_____

3. Today I am grateful for:
_____
_____
_____
_____

Day: _____   Date: __/__/___

1. Today's message to myself:

_____

2. Someone I could surprise with a note, gift or sign of appreciation and why:

_____

3. Today I am grateful for:

_____

_____

_____

_____

Day: _____   Date: __/__/___

1. Today's message to myself:

_____

2. Someone I could surprise with a note, gift or sign of appreciation and why:

_____

3. Today I am grateful for:

_____

_____

_____

_____

Day: _____   Date: __/__/___

1. Today's message to myself:

_____

2. Someone I could surprise with a note, gift or sign of appreciation and why:

_____

3. Today I am grateful for:

_____

_____

_____

_____

The future is today.
— William Osler

Day: _____   Date: __/__/____

1. Today's message to myself:

_____

2. Someone I could surprise with a note, gift or sign of appreciation and why:

_____

3. Today I am grateful for:

_____

_____

_____

_____

Day: _____   Date: __/__/____

1. Today's message to myself:

_____

2. Someone I could surprise with a note, gift or sign of appreciation and why:

_____

3. Today I am grateful for:

_____

_____

_____

_____

Day: _____   Date: __/__/____

1. Today's message to myself:

_____

2. Someone I could surprise with a note, gift or sign of appreciation and why:

_____

3. Today I am grateful for:

_____

_____

_____

_____

Day: _____   Date: __/__/____

1. Today's message to myself:

_____

2. Someone I could surprise with a note, gift or sign of appreciation and why:

_____

3. Today I am grateful for:

_____

_____

_____

_____

Day: _____   Date: __/__/____

1. Today's message to myself:

_____

2. Someone I could surprise with a note, gift or sign of appreciation and why:

_____

3. Today I am grateful for:

_____

_____

_____

_____

Day: _____   Date: __/__/____

1. Today's message to myself:

_____

2. Someone I could surprise with a note, gift or sign of appreciation and why:

_____

3. Today I am grateful for:

_____

_____

_____

_____

Our life always expresses the result of our dominant thoughts.
— Soren Kierkegaard

Day: _____   Date: _/_/___

1. Today's message to myself:

_____

2. Someone I could surprise with a note, gift or sign of appreciation and why:

_____

3. Today I am grateful for:

_____

_____

_____

_____

Day: _____   Date: _/_/___

1. Today's message to myself:

_____

2. Someone I could surprise with a note, gift or sign of appreciation and why:

_____

3. Today I am grateful for:

_____

_____

_____

_____

Day: _____   Date: _/_/___

1. Today's message to myself:

_____

2. Someone I could surprise with a note, gift or sign of appreciation and why:

_____

3. Today I am grateful for:

_____

_____

_____

The earth laughs in flowers.
— Ralph Waldo Emerson

Day: _____   Date: __/__/___

1. Today's message to myself:

_____

2. Someone I could surprise with a note, gift or sign of appreciation and why:

_____

3. Today I am grateful for:

_____

_____

_____

_____

Day: _____   Date: __/__/___

1. Today's message to myself:

_____

2. Someone I could surprise with a note, gift or sign of appreciation and why:

_____

3. Today I am grateful for:

_____

_____

_____

_____

Day: _____   Date: __/__/___

1. Today's message to myself:

_____

2. Someone I could surprise with a note, gift or sign of appreciation and why:

_____

3. Today I am grateful for:

_____

_____

_____

_____

Good actions give strength to ourselves and inspire good actions in others. — Plato

Day: _____   Date: __/__/___

1. Today's message to myself:

_____

2. Someone I could surprise with a note, gift or sign of appreciation and why:

_____

3. Today I am grateful for:

_____

_____

_____

_____

Day: _____   Date: __/__/___

1. Today's message to myself:

_____

2. Someone I could surprise with a note, gift or sign of appreciation and why:

_____

3. Today I am grateful for:

_____

_____

_____

_____

Day: _____   Date: __/__/___

1. Today's message to myself:

_____

2. Someone I could surprise with a note, gift or sign of appreciation and why:

_____

3. Today I am grateful for:

_____

_____

_____

Let the beauty of what you love be what you do.
— Rumi

Day: _____   Date: __/__/____

1. Today's message to myself:
_____

2. Someone I could surprise with a note, gift or sign of appreciation and why:
_____

3. Today I am grateful for:
_____
_____
_____
_____

Day: _____   Date: __/__/____

1. Today's message to myself:
_____

2. Someone I could surprise with a note, gift or sign of appreciation and why:
_____

3. Today I am grateful for:
_____
_____
_____
_____

Day: _____   Date: __/__/____

1. Today's message to myself:
_____

2. Someone I could surprise with a note, gift or sign of appreciation and why:
_____

3. Today I am grateful for:
_____
_____
_____
_____

Who seeks shall find.
— Sophocles

Day: _____   Date: __/__/____

1. Today's message to myself:

_____

2. Someone I could surprise with a note, gift or sign of appreciation and why:

_____

3. Today I am grateful for:

_____

_____

_____

Day: _____   Date: __/__/____

1. Today's message to myself:

_____

2. Someone I could surprise with a note, gift or sign of appreciation and why:

_____

3. Today I am grateful for:

_____

_____

_____

Day: _____   Date: __/__/____

1. Today's message to myself:

_____

2. Someone I could surprise with a note, gift or sign of appreciation and why:

_____

3. Today I am grateful for:

_____

_____

_____

Day: _____   Date: __/__/____

1. Today's message to myself:

_____

2. Someone I could surprise with a note, gift or sign of appreciation and why:

_____

3. Today I am grateful for:

_____

_____

_____

_____

Day: _____   Date: __/__/____

1. Today's message to myself:

_____

2. Someone I could surprise with a note, gift or sign of appreciation and why:

_____

3. Today I am grateful for:

_____

_____

_____

_____

Day: _____   Date: __/__/____

1. Today's message to myself:

_____

2. Someone I could surprise with a note, gift or sign of appreciation and why:

_____

3. Today I am grateful for:

_____

_____

_____

_____

The greatest weapon against stress is our ability to choose one
thought over another. — William James

Day: _____   Date: __/__/____

1. Today's message to myself:

_____

2. Someone I could surprise with a note, gift or sign of appreciation and why:

_____

3. Today I am grateful for:

_____

_____

_____

_____

Day: _____   Date: __/__/____

1. Today's message to myself:

_____

2. Someone I could surprise with a note, gift or sign of appreciation and why:

_____

3. Today I am grateful for:

_____

_____

_____

_____

Day: _____   Date: __/__/____

1. Today's message to myself:

_____

2. Someone I could surprise with a note, gift or sign of appreciation and why:

_____

3. Today I am grateful for:

_____

_____

_____

A Moment of Mindfulness

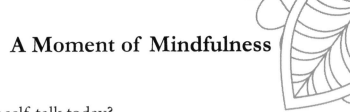

How is my self-talk today?

How is my body today?

What nourishes me?

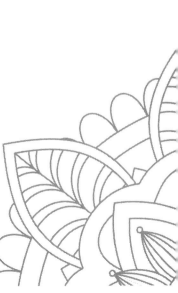

My life has been full of terrible misfortunes most of
which never happened. — Michel de Montaigne

Day: _____   Date: __/__/___

1. Today's message to myself:

_____

2. Someone I could surprise with a note, gift or sign of appreciation and why:

_____

3. Today I am grateful for:

_____

_____

_____

_____

Day: _____   Date: __/__/___

1. Today's message to myself:

_____

2. Someone I could surprise with a note, gift or sign of appreciation and why:

_____

3. Today I am grateful for:

_____

_____

_____

_____

Day: _____   Date: __/__/___

1. Today's message to myself:

_____

2. Someone I could surprise with a note, gift or sign of appreciation and why:

_____

3. Today I am grateful for:

_____

_____

_____

_____

When unhappy, one doubts everything; when happy,
one doubts nothing. — Joseph Roux

Day: _____   Date: __/__/___

1. Today's message to myself:
_____

2. Someone I could surprise with a note, gift or sign of appreciation and why:
_____

3. Today I am grateful for:
_____
_____
_____
_____

Day: _____   Date: __/__/___

1. Today's message to myself:
_____

2. Someone I could surprise with a note, gift or sign of appreciation and why:
_____

3. Today I am grateful for:
_____
_____
_____
_____

Day: _____   Date: __/__/___

1. Today's message to myself:
_____

2. Someone I could surprise with a note, gift or sign of appreciation and why:
_____

3. Today I am grateful for:
_____
_____
_____
_____

A single grateful thought toward heaven is the most perfect prayer.
— Gotthold Ephraim Lessing

Day: _____   Date: __/__/____

1. Today's message to myself:

_____

2. Someone I could surprise with a note, gift or sign of appreciation and why:

_____

3. Today I am grateful for:

_____
_____
_____
_____

Day: _____   Date: __/__/____

1. Today's message to myself:

_____

2. Someone I could surprise with a note, gift or sign of appreciation and why:

_____

3. Today I am grateful for:

_____
_____
_____
_____

Day: _____   Date: __/__/____

1. Today's message to myself:

_____

2. Someone I could surprise with a note, gift or sign of appreciation and why:

_____

3. Today I am grateful for:

_____
_____
_____
_____

When I let go of what I am, I become what I might be.
— Lao Tzu

Day: _____   Date: __/__/____

1. Today's message to myself:
_____

2. Someone I could surprise with a note, gift or sign of appreciation and why:
_____

3. Today I am grateful for:
_____
_____
_____

Day: _____   Date: __/__/____

1. Today's message to myself:
_____

2. Someone I could surprise with a note, gift or sign of appreciation and why:
_____

3. Today I am grateful for:
_____
_____
_____

Day: _____   Date: __/__/____

1. Today's message to myself:
_____

2. Someone I could surprise with a note, gift or sign of appreciation and why:
_____

3. Today I am grateful for:
_____
_____
_____

To live is so startling it leaves little time for anything else.
— Emily Dickinson

Day: _____   Date: __/__/____

1. Today's message to myself:

_____

2. Someone I could surprise with a note, gift or sign of appreciation and why:

_____

3. Today I am grateful for:

_____
_____
_____
_____

Day: _____   Date: __/__/____

1. Today's message to myself:

_____

2. Someone I could surprise with a note, gift or sign of appreciation and why:

_____

3. Today I am grateful for:

_____
_____
_____
_____

Day: _____   Date: __/__/____

1. Today's message to myself:

_____

2. Someone I could surprise with a note, gift or sign of appreciation and why:

_____

3. Today I am grateful for:

_____
_____
_____

Three grand essentials to happiness in this life are something to do, something to love, and something to hope for. — Joseph Addison

Day: _____   Date: __/__/__

1. Today's message to myself:

_____

2. Someone I could surprise with a note, gift or sign of appreciation and why:

_____

3. Today I am grateful for:

_____
_____
_____
_____

Day: _____   Date: __/__/__

1. Today's message to myself:

_____

2. Someone I could surprise with a note, gift or sign of appreciation and why:

_____

3. Today I am grateful for:

_____
_____
_____
_____

Day: _____   Date: __/__/__

1. Today's message to myself:

_____

2. Someone I could surprise with a note, gift or sign of appreciation and why:

_____

3. Today I am grateful for:

_____
_____
_____
_____

Keep your face always toward the sunshine - and shadows
will fall behind you. — Walt Whitman

Day: _____   Date: __/__/___

1. Today's message to myself:

_____

2. Someone I could surprise with a note, gift or sign of appreciation and why:

_____

3. Today I am grateful for:

_____

_____

_____

_____

Day: _____   Date: __/__/___

1. Today's message to myself:

_____

2. Someone I could surprise with a note, gift or sign of appreciation and why:

_____

3. Today I am grateful for:

_____

_____

_____

_____

Day: _____   Date: __/__/___

1. Today's message to myself:

_____

2. Someone I could surprise with a note, gift or sign of appreciation and why:

_____

3. Today I am grateful for:

_____

_____

_____

_____

> We love life, not because we are used to living but because
> we are used to loving. — Friedrich Nietzsche

Day: _____   Date: __/__/____

1. Today's message to myself:
_____

2. Someone I could surprise with a note, gift or sign of appreciation and why:
_____

3. Today I am grateful for:
_____
_____
_____
_____

Day: _____   Date: __/__/____

1. Today's message to myself:
_____

2. Someone I could surprise with a note, gift or sign of appreciation and why:
_____

3. Today I am grateful for:
_____
_____
_____
_____

Day: _____   Date: __/__/____

1. Today's message to myself:
_____

2. Someone I could surprise with a note, gift or sign of appreciation and why:
_____

3. Today I am grateful for:
_____
_____
_____

True originality consists not in a new manner but in a new vision.
— Edith Wharton

Day: _____   Date: __/__/____

1. Today's message to myself:

_____

2. Someone I could surprise with a note, gift or sign of appreciation and why:

_____

3. Today I am grateful for:

_____

_____

_____

_____

Day: _____   Date: __/__/____

1. Today's message to myself:

_____

2. Someone I could surprise with a note, gift or sign of appreciation and why:

_____

3. Today I am grateful for:

_____

_____

_____

_____

Day: _____   Date: __/__/____

1. Today's message to myself:

_____

2. Someone I could surprise with a note, gift or sign of appreciation and why:

_____

3. Today I am grateful for:

_____

_____

_____

_____

The best part of beauty is that which no picture can express.
— Francis Bacon

Day: _____   Date: __/__/___

1. Today's message to myself:
_____

2. Someone I could surprise with a note, gift or sign of appreciation and why:
_____

3. Today I am grateful for:
_____
_____
_____
_____

Day: _____   Date: __/__/___

1. Today's message to myself:
_____

2. Someone I could surprise with a note, gift or sign of appreciation and why:
_____

3. Today I am grateful for:
_____
_____
_____
_____

Day: _____   Date: __/__/___

1. Today's message to myself:
_____

2. Someone I could surprise with a note, gift or sign of appreciation and why:
_____

3. Today I am grateful for:
_____
_____
_____
_____

The things that we love tell us what we are.
— Thomas Aquinas

Day: _____   Date: __/__/____

1. Today's message to myself:

_____

2. Someone I could surprise with a note, gift or sign of appreciation and why:

_____

3. Today I am grateful for:

_____
_____
_____
_____

Day: _____   Date: __/__/____

1. Today's message to myself:

_____

2. Someone I could surprise with a note, gift or sign of appreciation and why:

_____

3. Today I am grateful for:

_____
_____
_____
_____

Day: _____   Date: __/__/____

1. Today's message to myself:

_____

2. Someone I could surprise with a note, gift or sign of appreciation and why:

_____

3. Today I am grateful for:

_____
_____
_____

One that would have the fruit must climb the tree.
— Thomas Fuller

Day: _____   Date: __/__/____

1. Today's message to myself:
_____

2. Someone I could surprise with a note, gift or sign of appreciation and why:
_____

3. Today I am grateful for:
_____
_____
_____
_____

Day: _____   Date: __/__/____

1. Today's message to myself:
_____

2. Someone I could surprise with a note, gift or sign of appreciation and why:
_____

3. Today I am grateful for:
_____
_____
_____
_____

Day: _____   Date: __/__/____

1. Today's message to myself:
_____

2. Someone I could surprise with a note, gift or sign of appreciation and why:
_____

3. Today I am grateful for:
_____
_____
_____

We do not see nature with our eyes, but with our understandings and our hearts. — William Hazlitt

Day: _____   Date: _/_/____

1. Today's message to myself:

_____

2. Someone I could surprise with a note, gift or sign of appreciation and why:

_____

3. Today I am grateful for:

_____

_____

_____

_____

Day: _____   Date: _/_/____

1. Today's message to myself:

_____

2. Someone I could surprise with a note, gift or sign of appreciation and why:

_____

3. Today I am grateful for:

_____

_____

_____

_____

Day: _____   Date: _/_/____

1. Today's message to myself:

_____

2. Someone I could surprise with a note, gift or sign of appreciation and why:

_____

3. Today I am grateful for:

_____

_____

_____

A Moment of Mindfulness

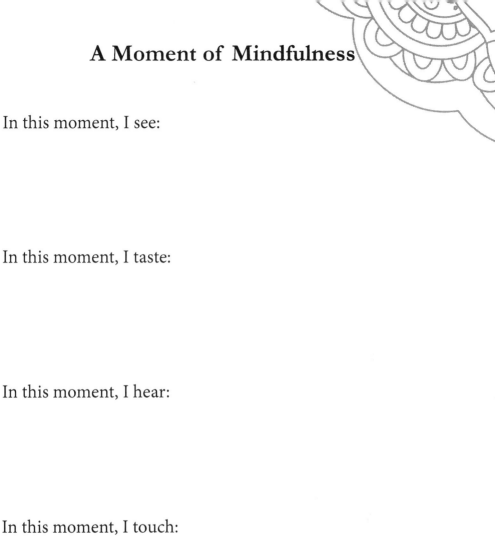

In this moment, I see:

In this moment, I taste:

In this moment, I hear:

In this moment, I touch:

In this moment, I smell:

For the will and not the gift makes the giver.
— Gotthold Ephraim Lessing

Day: _____   Date: __/__/____

1. Today's message to myself:

_____

2. Someone I could surprise with a note, gift or sign of appreciation and why:

_____

3. Today I am grateful for:

_____

_____

_____

_____

Day: _____   Date: __/__/____

1. Today's message to myself:

_____

2. Someone I could surprise with a note, gift or sign of appreciation and why:

_____

3. Today I am grateful for:

_____

_____

_____

_____

Day: _____   Date: __/__/____

1. Today's message to myself:

_____

2. Someone I could surprise with a note, gift or sign of appreciation and why:

_____

3. Today I am grateful for:

_____

_____

_____

_____

Beauty is not caused. It is.
— Emily Dickinson

Day: _____   Date: _/_/____

1. Today's message to myself:

_____

2. Someone I could surprise with a note, gift or sign of appreciation and why:

_____

3. Today I am grateful for:

_____

_____

_____

_____

Day: _____   Date: _/_/____

1. Today's message to myself:

_____

2. Someone I could surprise with a note, gift or sign of appreciation and why:

_____

3. Today I am grateful for:

_____

_____

_____

_____

Day: _____   Date: _/_/____

1. Today's message to myself:

_____

2. Someone I could surprise with a note, gift or sign of appreciation and why:

_____

3. Today I am grateful for:

_____

_____

_____

_____

Happiness is not an ideal of reason, but of imagination.
— Immanuel Kant

Day: _____   Date: _/_/___

1. Today's message to myself:

2. Someone I could surprise with a note, gift or sign of appreciation and why:

3. Today I am grateful for:

Day: _____   Date: _/_/___

1. Today's message to myself:

2. Someone I could surprise with a note, gift or sign of appreciation and why:

3. Today I am grateful for:

Day: _____   Date: _/_/___

1. Today's message to myself:

2. Someone I could surprise with a note, gift or sign of appreciation and why:

3. Today I am grateful for:

There is nothing that makes its way more directly into the
soul than beauty. — Joseph Addison

Day: _____   Date: __/__/____

1. Today's message to myself:

_____

2. Someone I could surprise with a note, gift or sign of appreciation and why:

_____

3. Today I am grateful for:

_____

_____

_____

_____

Day: _____   Date: __/__/____

1. Today's message to myself:

_____

2. Someone I could surprise with a note, gift or sign of appreciation and why:

_____

3. Today I am grateful for:

_____

_____

_____

_____

Day: _____   Date: __/__/____

1. Today's message to myself:

_____

2. Someone I could surprise with a note, gift or sign of appreciation and why:

_____

3. Today I am grateful for:

_____

_____

_____

_____

Do exactly what you would do if you felt most secure.
— Meister Eckhart

Day: _____   Date: __/__/____

1. Today's message to myself:

_____

2. Someone I could surprise with a note, gift or sign of appreciation and why:

_____

3. Today I am grateful for:

_____

_____

_____

_____

Day: _____   Date: __/__/____

1. Today's message to myself:

_____

2. Someone I could surprise with a note, gift or sign of appreciation and why:

_____

3. Today I am grateful for:

_____

_____

_____

_____

Day: _____   Date: __/__/____

1. Today's message to myself:

_____

2. Someone I could surprise with a note, gift or sign of appreciation and why:

_____

3. Today I am grateful for:

_____

_____

_____

_____

Let each become all that he was created capable of being.
— Thomas Carlyle

Day: _____   Date: __/__/___

1. Today's message to myself:
_____

2. Someone I could surprise with a note, gift or sign of appreciation and why:
_____

3. Today I am grateful for:
_____
_____
_____
_____

Day: _____   Date: __/__/___

1. Today's message to myself:
_____

2. Someone I could surprise with a note, gift or sign of appreciation and why:
_____

3. Today I am grateful for:
_____
_____
_____
_____

Day: _____   Date: __/__/___

1. Today's message to myself:
_____

2. Someone I could surprise with a note, gift or sign of appreciation and why:
_____

3. Today I am grateful for:
_____
_____
_____
_____

Time is flying never to return.
— Virgil

Day: _____   Date: __/__/____

1. Today's message to myself:
_____

2. Someone I could surprise with a note, gift or sign of appreciation and why:
_____

3. Today I am grateful for:
_____
_____
_____
_____

Day: _____   Date: __/__/____

1. Today's message to myself:
_____

2. Someone I could surprise with a note, gift or sign of appreciation and why:
_____

3. Today I am grateful for:
_____
_____
_____
_____

Day: _____   Date: __/__/____

1. Today's message to myself:
_____

2. Someone I could surprise with a note, gift or sign of appreciation and why:
_____

3. Today I am grateful for:
_____
_____
_____

It does not matter how slowly you go as long as you do not stop.
— Confucius

Day: _____   Date: _/_/___

1. Today's message to myself:
_____

2. Someone I could surprise with a note, gift or sign of appreciation and why:
_____

3. Today I am grateful for:
_____
_____
_____
_____

Day: _____   Date: _/_/___

1. Today's message to myself:
_____

2. Someone I could surprise with a note, gift or sign of appreciation and why:
_____

3. Today I am grateful for:
_____
_____
_____
_____

Day: _____   Date: _/_/___

1. Today's message to myself:
_____

2. Someone I could surprise with a note, gift or sign of appreciation and why:
_____

3. Today I am grateful for:
_____
_____
_____
_____

The journey of a thousand miles begins with one step.
— Lao Tzu

Day: _____   Date: __/__/____

1. Today's message to myself:

_____

2. Someone I could surprise with a note, gift or sign of appreciation and why:

_____

3. Today I am grateful for:

_____

_____

_____

_____

Day: _____   Date: __/__/____

1. Today's message to myself:

_____

2. Someone I could surprise with a note, gift or sign of appreciation and why:

_____

3. Today I am grateful for:

_____

_____

_____

_____

Day: _____   Date: __/__/____

1. Today's message to myself:

_____

2. Someone I could surprise with a note, gift or sign of appreciation and why:

_____

3. Today I am grateful for:

_____

_____

_____

_____

When I give I give myself.
— Walt Whitman

Day: _____   Date: __/__/____

1. Today's message to myself:
_____

2. Someone I could surprise with a note, gift or sign of appreciation and why:
_____

3. Today I am grateful for:
_____
_____
_____
_____

Day: _____   Date: __/__/____

1. Today's message to myself:
_____

2. Someone I could surprise with a note, gift or sign of appreciation and why:
_____

3. Today I am grateful for:
_____
_____
_____
_____

Day: _____   Date: __/__/____

1. Today's message to myself:
_____

2. Someone I could surprise with a note, gift or sign of appreciation and why:
_____

3. Today I am grateful for:
_____
_____
_____

Happiness is a virtue, not its reward.
— Baruch Spinoza

Day: _____   Date: __/__/___

1. Today's message to myself:

_____

2. Someone I could surprise with a note, gift or sign of appreciation and why:

_____

3. Today I am grateful for:

_____

_____

_____

_____

Day: _____   Date: __/__/___

1. Today's message to myself:

_____

2. Someone I could surprise with a note, gift or sign of appreciation and why:

_____

3. Today I am grateful for:

_____

_____

_____

_____

Day: _____   Date: __/__/___

1. Today's message to myself:

_____

2. Someone I could surprise with a note, gift or sign of appreciation and why:

_____

3. Today I am grateful for:

_____

_____

_____

_____

It's easier to go down a hill than up it but the view is much
better at the top. — Henry Ward Beecher

Day: _____   Date: __/__/___

1. Today's message to myself:
_____

2. Someone I could surprise with a note, gift or sign of appreciation and why:
_____

3. Today I am grateful for:
_____
_____
_____
_____

Day: _____   Date: __/__/___

1. Today's message to myself:
_____

2. Someone I could surprise with a note, gift or sign of appreciation and why:
_____

3. Today I am grateful for:
_____
_____
_____
_____

Day: _____   Date: __/__/___

1. Today's message to myself:
_____

2. Someone I could surprise with a note, gift or sign of appreciation and why:
_____

3. Today I am grateful for:
_____
_____
_____

A friend is a gift you give yourself.
— Robert Louis Stevenson

Day: _____   Date: __/__/____

1. Today's message to myself:

_____

2. Someone I could surprise with a note, gift or sign of appreciation and why:

_____

3. Today I am grateful for:

_____

_____

_____

_____

Day: _____   Date: __/__/____

1. Today's message to myself:

_____

2. Someone I could surprise with a note, gift or sign of appreciation and why:

_____

3. Today I am grateful for:

_____

_____

_____

_____

Day: _____   Date: __/__/____

1. Today's message to myself:

_____

2. Someone I could surprise with a note, gift or sign of appreciation and why:

_____

3. Today I am grateful for:

_____

_____

_____

_____

A Moment of Mindfulness

I commit to:

I affirm:

I intend:

Lend yourself to others, but give yourself to yourself.
— Michel de Montaigne

Day: _____   Date: __/__/___

1. Today's message to myself:
_____

2. Someone I could surprise with a note, gift or sign of appreciation and why:
_____

3. Today I am grateful for:
_____
_____
_____
_____

Day: _____   Date: __/__/___

1. Today's message to myself:
_____

2. Someone I could surprise with a note, gift or sign of appreciation and why:
_____

3. Today I am grateful for:
_____
_____
_____
_____

Day: _____   Date: __/__/___

1. Today's message to myself:
_____

2. Someone I could surprise with a note, gift or sign of appreciation and why:
_____

3. Today I am grateful for:
_____
_____
_____

Keep love in your heart. A life without it is like a sunless garden
when the flowers are dead. — Oscar Wilde

Day: _____   Date: __/__/___

1. Today's message to myself:
_____

2. Someone I could surprise with a note, gift or sign of appreciation and why:
_____

3. Today I am grateful for:
_____
_____
_____
_____

Day: _____   Date: __/__/___

1. Today's message to myself:
_____

2. Someone I could surprise with a note, gift or sign of appreciation and why:
_____

3. Today I am grateful for:
_____
_____
_____
_____

Day: _____   Date: __/__/___

1. Today's message to myself:
_____

2. Someone I could surprise with a note, gift or sign of appreciation and why:
_____

3. Today I am grateful for:
_____
_____
_____

Be content with your lot; one cannot be first in everything.
— Aesop

Day: _____   Date: __/__/____

1. Today's message to myself:

_____

2. Someone I could surprise with a note, gift or sign of appreciation and why:

_____

3. Today I am grateful for:

_____

_____

_____

_____

Day: _____   Date: __/__/____

1. Today's message to myself:

_____

2. Someone I could surprise with a note, gift or sign of appreciation and why:

_____

3. Today I am grateful for:

_____

_____

_____

_____

Day: _____   Date: __/__/____

1. Today's message to myself:

_____

2. Someone I could surprise with a note, gift or sign of appreciation and why:

_____

3. Today I am grateful for:

_____

_____

_____

_____

In character, in manner, in style, in all things, the supreme excellence is simplicity. — Henry Wadsworth Longfellow

Day: _____   Date: __/__/____

1. Today's message to myself:
_____

2. Someone I could surprise with a note, gift or sign of appreciation and why:
_____

3. Today I am grateful for:
_____
_____
_____
_____

Day: _____   Date: __/__/____

1. Today's message to myself:
_____

2. Someone I could surprise with a note, gift or sign of appreciation and why:
_____

3. Today I am grateful for:
_____
_____
_____
_____

Day: _____   Date: __/__/____

1. Today's message to myself:
_____

2. Someone I could surprise with a note, gift or sign of appreciation and why:
_____

3. Today I am grateful for:
_____
_____
_____

What we achieve inwardly will change outer reality.
— Plutarch

Day: _____   Date: __/__/___

1. Today's message to myself:

_____

2. Someone I could surprise with a note, gift or sign of appreciation and why:

_____

3. Today I am grateful for:

_____

_____

_____

_____

Day: _____   Date: __/__/___

1. Today's message to myself:

_____

2. Someone I could surprise with a note, gift or sign of appreciation and why:

_____

3. Today I am grateful for:

_____

_____

_____

_____

Day: _____   Date: __/__/___

1. Today's message to myself:

_____

2. Someone I could surprise with a note, gift or sign of appreciation and why:

_____

3. Today I am grateful for:

_____

_____

_____

That man is a success who has lived well, laughed often and
loved much. — Robert Louis Stevenson

Day: _____   Date: __/__/___

1. Today's message to myself:

_____

2. Someone I could surprise with a note, gift or sign of appreciation and why:

_____

3. Today I am grateful for:

_____

_____

_____

_____

Day: _____   Date: __/__/___

1. Today's message to myself:

_____

2. Someone I could surprise with a note, gift or sign of appreciation and why:

_____

3. Today I am grateful for:

_____

_____

_____

_____

Day: _____   Date: __/__/___

1. Today's message to myself:

_____

2. Someone I could surprise with a note, gift or sign of appreciation and why:

_____

3. Today I am grateful for:

_____

_____

_____

_____

The key is to keep company only with people who uplift you, whose presence calls forth your best. — Epictetus

Day: _____   Date: __/__/____

1. Today's message to myself:

2. Someone I could surprise with a note, gift or sign of appreciation and why:

3. Today I am grateful for:

Day: _____   Date: __/__/____

1. Today's message to myself:

2. Someone I could surprise with a note, gift or sign of appreciation and why:

3. Today I am grateful for:

Day: _____   Date: __/__/____

1. Today's message to myself:

2. Someone I could surprise with a note, gift or sign of appreciation and why:

3. Today I am grateful for:

Day: _____   Date: __/__/___

1. Today's message to myself:

_____

2. Someone I could surprise with a note, gift or sign of appreciation and why:

_____

3. Today I am grateful for:

_____

_____

_____

_____

Day: _____   Date: __/__/___

1. Today's message to myself:

_____

2. Someone I could surprise with a note, gift or sign of appreciation and why:

_____

3. Today I am grateful for:

_____

_____

_____

_____

Day: _____   Date: __/__/___

1. Today's message to myself:

_____

2. Someone I could surprise with a note, gift or sign of appreciation and why:

_____

3. Today I am grateful for:

_____

_____

_____

Persevere and preserve yourselves for better circumstances.
— Virgil

Day: _____   Date: __/__/___

1. Today's message to myself:

_____

2. Someone I could surprise with a note, gift or sign of appreciation and why:

_____

3. Today I am grateful for:

_____

_____

_____

_____

Day: _____   Date: __/__/___

1. Today's message to myself:

_____

2. Someone I could surprise with a note, gift or sign of appreciation and why:

_____

3. Today I am grateful for:

_____

_____

_____

_____

Day: _____   Date: __/__/___

1. Today's message to myself:

_____

2. Someone I could surprise with a note, gift or sign of appreciation and why:

_____

3. Today I am grateful for:

_____

_____

_____

_____

> Think for yourselves and let others enjoy the privilege to do so, too.
> — Voltaire

Day: _____   Date: __/__/____

1. Today's message to myself:
_____

2. Someone I could surprise with a note, gift or sign of appreciation and why:
_____

3. Today I am grateful for:
_____
_____
_____
_____

Day: _____   Date: __/__/____

1. Today's message to myself:
_____

2. Someone I could surprise with a note, gift or sign of appreciation and why:
_____

3. Today I am grateful for:
_____
_____
_____
_____

Day: _____   Date: __/__/____

1. Today's message to myself:
_____

2. Someone I could surprise with a note, gift or sign of appreciation and why:
_____

3. Today I am grateful for:
_____
_____
_____

Wherever you go, go with all your heart.
— Confucius

Day: _____   Date: __/__/___

1. Today's message to myself:

_____

2. Someone I could surprise with a note, gift or sign of appreciation and why:

_____

3. Today I am grateful for:

_____

_____

_____

_____

Day: _____   Date: __/__/___

1. Today's message to myself:

_____

2. Someone I could surprise with a note, gift or sign of appreciation and why:

_____

3. Today I am grateful for:

_____

_____

_____

_____

Day: _____   Date: __/__/___

1. Today's message to myself:

_____

2. Someone I could surprise with a note, gift or sign of appreciation and why:

_____

3. Today I am grateful for:

_____

_____

_____

_____

The sun does not shine for a few trees and flowers, but for the
wide world's joy. — Henry Ward Beecher

Day: _____   Date: __/__/___

1. Today's message to myself:
_____

2. Someone I could surprise with a note, gift or sign of appreciation and why:
_____

3. Today I am grateful for:
_____
_____
_____
_____

Day: _____   Date: __/__/___

1. Today's message to myself:
_____

2. Someone I could surprise with a note, gift or sign of appreciation and why:
_____

3. Today I am grateful for:
_____
_____
_____
_____

Day: _____   Date: __/__/___

1. Today's message to myself:
_____

2. Someone I could surprise with a note, gift or sign of appreciation and why:
_____

3. Today I am grateful for:
_____
_____
_____

Fear cannot be without hope nor hope without fear.
— Baruch Spinoza

Day: _____   Date: __/__/___

1. Today's message to myself:
_____

2. Someone I could surprise with a note, gift or sign of appreciation and why:
_____

3. Today I am grateful for:
_____
_____
_____
_____

Day: _____   Date: __/__/___

1. Today's message to myself:
_____

2. Someone I could surprise with a note, gift or sign of appreciation and why:
_____

3. Today I am grateful for:
_____
_____
_____
_____

Day: _____   Date: __/__/___

1. Today's message to myself:
_____

2. Someone I could surprise with a note, gift or sign of appreciation and why:
_____

3. Today I am grateful for:
_____
_____
_____

A Moment of Mindfulness

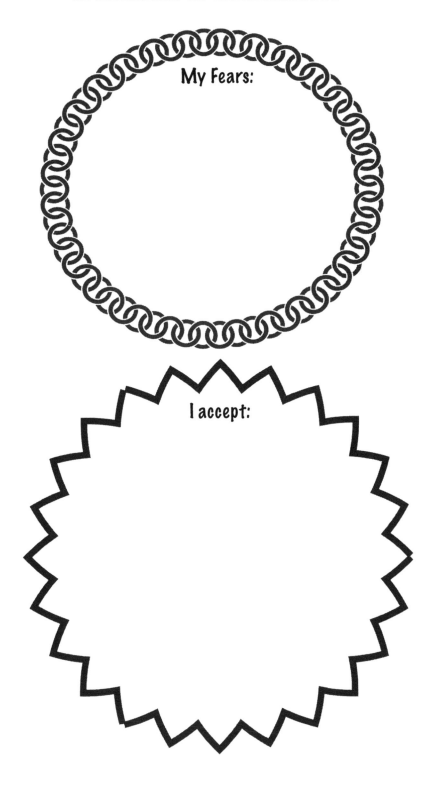

My Fears:

I accept:

The energy of the mind is the essence of life.
— Aristotle

Day: _____   Date: __/__/____

1. Today's message to myself:

_____

2. Someone I could surprise with a note, gift or sign of appreciation and why:

_____

3. Today I am grateful for:

_____

_____

_____

_____

Day: _____   Date: __/__/____

1. Today's message to myself:

_____

2. Someone I could surprise with a note, gift or sign of appreciation and why:

_____

3. Today I am grateful for:

_____

_____

_____

_____

Day: _____   Date: __/__/____

1. Today's message to myself:

_____

2. Someone I could surprise with a note, gift or sign of appreciation and why:

_____

3. Today I am grateful for:

_____

_____

_____

_____

The happiness which is lacking makes one think even the
happiness one has unbearable. — Joseph Roux

Day: _____   Date: __/__/____

1. Today's message to myself:
_____

2. Someone I could surprise with a note, gift or sign of appreciation and why:
_____

3. Today I am grateful for:
_____
_____
_____
_____

Day: _____   Date: __/__/____

1. Today's message to myself:
_____

2. Someone I could surprise with a note, gift or sign of appreciation and why:
_____

3. Today I am grateful for:
_____
_____
_____
_____

Day: _____   Date: __/__/____

1. Today's message to myself:
_____

2. Someone I could surprise with a note, gift or sign of appreciation and why:
_____

3. Today I am grateful for:
_____
_____
_____

For every minute you remain angry, you give up sixty seconds
of peace of mind. — Ralph Waldo Emerson

Day: _____   Date: __/__/___

1. Today's message to myself:

_____

2. Someone I could surprise with a note, gift or sign of appreciation and why:

_____

3. Today I am grateful for:

_____
_____
_____
_____

Day: _____   Date: __/__/___

1. Today's message to myself:

_____

2. Someone I could surprise with a note, gift or sign of appreciation and why:

_____

3. Today I am grateful for:

_____
_____
_____
_____

Day: _____   Date: __/__/___

1. Today's message to myself:

_____

2. Someone I could surprise with a note, gift or sign of appreciation and why:

_____

3. Today I am grateful for:

_____
_____
_____
_____

Love takes up where knowledge leaves off.
— Thomas Aquinas

Day: _____   Date: _/_/___

1. Today's message to myself:
_____

2. Someone I could surprise with a note, gift or sign of appreciation and why:
_____

3. Today I am grateful for:
_____
_____
_____
_____

Day: _____   Date: _/_/___

1. Today's message to myself:
_____

2. Someone I could surprise with a note, gift or sign of appreciation and why:
_____

3. Today I am grateful for:
_____
_____
_____
_____

Day: _____   Date: _/_/___

1. Today's message to myself:
_____

2. Someone I could surprise with a note, gift or sign of appreciation and why:
_____

3. Today I am grateful for:
_____
_____
_____
_____

Our life is what our thoughts make it.
— Marcus Aurelius

Day: _____   Date: __/__/___

1. Today's message to myself:

_____

2. Someone I could surprise with a note, gift or sign of appreciation and why:

_____

3. Today I am grateful for:

_____

_____

_____

_____

Day: _____   Date: __/__/___

1. Today's message to myself:

_____

2. Someone I could surprise with a note, gift or sign of appreciation and why:

_____

3. Today I am grateful for:

_____

_____

_____

_____

Day: _____   Date: __/__/___

1. Today's message to myself:

_____

2. Someone I could surprise with a note, gift or sign of appreciation and why:

_____

3. Today I am grateful for:

_____

_____

_____

_____

Write it on your heart that every day is the best day in the year.
— Ralph Waldo Emerson

Day: _____   Date: __/__/____

1. Today's message to myself:

_____

2. Someone I could surprise with a note, gift or sign of appreciation and why:

_____

3. Today I am grateful for:

_____

_____

_____

_____

Day: _____   Date: __/__/____

1. Today's message to myself:

_____

2. Someone I could surprise with a note, gift or sign of appreciation and why:

_____

3. Today I am grateful for:

_____

_____

_____

_____

Day: _____   Date: __/__/____

1. Today's message to myself:

_____

2. Someone I could surprise with a note, gift or sign of appreciation and why:

_____

3. Today I am grateful for:

_____

_____

_____

_____

When the mind is thinking it is talking to itself.
— Plato

Day: _____   Date: __/__/___

1. Today's message to myself:

_____

2. Someone I could surprise with a note, gift or sign of appreciation and why:

_____

3. Today I am grateful for:

_____

_____

_____

_____

Day: _____   Date: __/__/___

1. Today's message to myself:

_____

2. Someone I could surprise with a note, gift or sign of appreciation and why:

_____

3. Today I am grateful for:

_____

_____

_____

_____

Day: _____   Date: __/__/___

1. Today's message to myself:

_____

2. Someone I could surprise with a note, gift or sign of appreciation and why:

_____

3. Today I am grateful for:

_____

_____

_____

_____

Day: _____   Date: __/__/____

1. Today's message to myself:

_____

2. Someone I could surprise with a note, gift or sign of appreciation and why:

_____

3. Today I am grateful for:

_____

_____

_____

_____

Day: _____   Date: __/__/____

1. Today's message to myself:

_____

2. Someone I could surprise with a note, gift or sign of appreciation and why:

_____

3. Today I am grateful for:

_____

_____

_____

_____

Day: _____   Date: __/__/____

1. Today's message to myself:

_____

2. Someone I could surprise with a note, gift or sign of appreciation and why:

_____

3. Today I am grateful for:

_____

_____

_____

_____

No act of kindness, no matter how small, is ever wasted.
— Aesop

Day: _____   Date: _/_/___

1. Today's message to myself:

_____

2. Someone I could surprise with a note, gift or sign of appreciation and why:

_____

3. Today I am grateful for:

_____

_____

_____

_____

Day: _____   Date: _/_/___

1. Today's message to myself:

_____

2. Someone I could surprise with a note, gift or sign of appreciation and why:

_____

3. Today I am grateful for:

_____

_____

_____

_____

Day: _____   Date: _/_/___

1. Today's message to myself:

_____

2. Someone I could surprise with a note, gift or sign of appreciation and why:

_____

3. Today I am grateful for:

_____

_____

_____

_____

If only we'd stop trying to be happy we'd have a pretty good time.
— Edith Wharton

Day: _____   Date: __/__/___

1. Today's message to myself:

_____

2. Someone I could surprise with a note, gift or sign of appreciation and why:

_____

3. Today I am grateful for:

_____

_____

_____

Day: _____   Date: __/__/___

1. Today's message to myself:

_____

2. Someone I could surprise with a note, gift or sign of appreciation and why:

_____

3. Today I am grateful for:

_____

_____

_____

_____

Day: _____   Date: __/__/___

1. Today's message to myself:

_____

2. Someone I could surprise with a note, gift or sign of appreciation and why:

_____

3. Today I am grateful for:

_____

_____

_____

There is only one way to happiness and that is to cease worrying about things which are beyond the power of our will. — Epictetus

Day: _____   Date: __/__/___

1. Today's message to myself:

_____

2. Someone I could surprise with a note, gift or sign of appreciation and why:

_____

3. Today I am grateful for:

_____

_____

_____

_____

Day: _____   Date: __/__/___

1. Today's message to myself:

_____

2. Someone I could surprise with a note, gift or sign of appreciation and why:

_____

3. Today I am grateful for:

_____

_____

_____

_____

Day: _____   Date: __/__/___

1. Today's message to myself:

_____

2. Someone I could surprise with a note, gift or sign of appreciation and why:

_____

3. Today I am grateful for:

_____

_____

_____

_____

The essence of all beautiful art, all great art, is gratitude.
— Friedrich Nietzsche

Day: _____   Date: __/__/___

1. Today's message to myself:
_____

2. Someone I could surprise with a note, gift or sign of appreciation and why:
_____

3. Today I am grateful for:
_____
_____
_____
_____

Day: _____   Date: __/__/___

1. Today's message to myself:
_____

2. Someone I could surprise with a note, gift or sign of appreciation and why:
_____

3. Today I am grateful for:
_____
_____
_____
_____

Day: _____   Date: __/__/___

1. Today's message to myself:
_____

2. Someone I could surprise with a note, gift or sign of appreciation and why:
_____

3. Today I am grateful for:
_____
_____
_____
_____

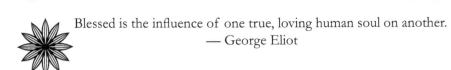

Blessed is the influence of one true, loving human soul on another.
— George Eliot

Day: _____   Date: __/__/___

1. Today's message to myself:

_____

2. Someone I could surprise with a note, gift or sign of appreciation and why:

_____

3. Today I am grateful for:

_____

_____

_____

_____

Day: _____   Date: __/__/___

1. Today's message to myself:

_____

2. Someone I could surprise with a note, gift or sign of appreciation and why:

_____

3. Today I am grateful for:

_____

_____

_____

_____

Day: _____   Date: __/__/___

1. Today's message to myself:

_____

2. Someone I could surprise with a note, gift or sign of appreciation and why:

_____

3. Today I am grateful for:

_____

_____

_____

A Moment of Mindfulness

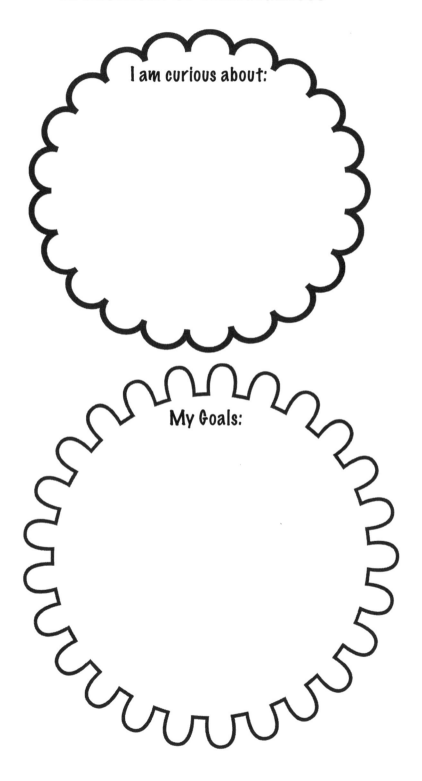

I am curious about:

My Goals:

For me the greatest beauty always lies in the greatest clarity.
— Gotthold Ephraim Lessing

Day: _____   Date: __/__/____

1. Today's message to myself:

_____

2. Someone I could surprise with a note, gift or sign of appreciation and why:

_____

3. Today I am grateful for:

_____

_____

_____

_____

Day: _____   Date: __/__/____

1. Today's message to myself:

_____

2. Someone I could surprise with a note, gift or sign of appreciation and why:

_____

3. Today I am grateful for:

_____

_____

_____

_____

Day: _____   Date: __/__/____

1. Today's message to myself:

_____

2. Someone I could surprise with a note, gift or sign of appreciation and why:

_____

3. Today I am grateful for:

_____

_____

_____

_____

Live your life as though your every act were to become a universal law.
— Immanuel Kant

Day: _____   Date: __/__/___

1. Today's message to myself:
_____

2. Someone I could surprise with a note, gift or sign of appreciation and why:
_____

3. Today I am grateful for:
_____
_____
_____
_____

Day: _____   Date: __/__/___

1. Today's message to myself:
_____

2. Someone I could surprise with a note, gift or sign of appreciation and why:
_____

3. Today I am grateful for:
_____
_____
_____
_____

Day: _____   Date: __/__/___

1. Today's message to myself:
_____

2. Someone I could surprise with a note, gift or sign of appreciation and why:
_____

3. Today I am grateful for:
_____
_____
_____

In every walk with nature one receives far more than he seeks.
— John Muir

Day: _____   Date: __/__/___

1. Today's message to myself:

_____

2. Someone I could surprise with a note, gift or sign of appreciation and why:

_____

3. Today I am grateful for:

_____

_____

_____

_____

Day: _____   Date: __/__/___

1. Today's message to myself:

_____

2. Someone I could surprise with a note, gift or sign of appreciation and why:

_____

3. Today I am grateful for:

_____

_____

_____

_____

Day: _____   Date: __/__/___

1. Today's message to myself:

_____

2. Someone I could surprise with a note, gift or sign of appreciation and why:

_____

3. Today I am grateful for:

_____

_____

_____

_____

Cheerfulness is the best promoter of health and is as friendly to the mind as to the body. — Joseph Addison

Day: _____　　　　　　　　Date: __/__/___

1. Today's message to myself:

_____

2. Someone I could surprise with a note, gift or sign of appreciation and why:

_____

3. Today I am grateful for:

_____

_____

_____

Day: _____　　　　　　　　Date: __/__/___

1. Today's message to myself:

_____

2. Someone I could surprise with a note, gift or sign of appreciation and why:

_____

3. Today I am grateful for:

_____

_____

_____

_____

Day: _____　　　　　　　　Date: __/__/___

1. Today's message to myself:

_____

2. Someone I could surprise with a note, gift or sign of appreciation and why:

_____

3. Today I am grateful for:

_____

_____

_____

He who knows others is wise. He who knows himself
is enlightened. — Lao Tzu

Day: _____   Date: __/__/___

1. Today's message to myself:

_____

2. Someone I could surprise with a note, gift or sign of appreciation and why:

_____

3. Today I am grateful for:

_____

_____

_____

_____

Day: _____   Date: __/__/___

1. Today's message to myself:

_____

2. Someone I could surprise with a note, gift or sign of appreciation and why:

_____

3. Today I am grateful for:

_____

_____

_____

_____

Day: _____   Date: __/__/___

1. Today's message to myself:

_____

2. Someone I could surprise with a note, gift or sign of appreciation and why:

_____

3. Today I am grateful for:

_____

_____

_____

_____

If the only prayer you ever say in your entire life is thank you,
it will be enough. — Meister Eckhart

Day: _____   Date: __/__/___

1. Today's message to myself:
_____

2. Someone I could surprise with a note, gift or sign of appreciation and why:
_____

3. Today I am grateful for:
_____
_____
_____
_____

Day: _____   Date: __/__/___

1. Today's message to myself:
_____

2. Someone I could surprise with a note, gift or sign of appreciation and why:
_____

3. Today I am grateful for:
_____
_____
_____
_____

Day: _____   Date: __/__/___

1. Today's message to myself:
_____

2. Someone I could surprise with a note, gift or sign of appreciation and why:
_____

3. Today I am grateful for:
_____
_____
_____
_____

Always forgive your enemies - nothing annoys them so much.
— Oscar Wilde

Day: _____   Date: _/_/___

1. Today's message to myself:

_____

2. Someone I could surprise with a note, gift or sign of appreciation and why:

_____

3. Today I am grateful for:

_____

_____

_____

_____

Day: _____   Date: _/_/___

1. Today's message to myself:

_____

2. Someone I could surprise with a note, gift or sign of appreciation and why:

_____

3. Today I am grateful for:

_____

_____

_____

_____

Day: _____   Date: _/_/___

1. Today's message to myself:

_____

2. Someone I could surprise with a note, gift or sign of appreciation and why:

_____

3. Today I am grateful for:

_____

_____

_____

_____

Don't grieve. Anything you lose comes round in another form.
— Rumi

Day: _____   Date: __/__/___

1. Today's message to myself:
_____

2. Someone I could surprise with a note, gift or sign of appreciation and why:
_____

3. Today I am grateful for:
_____
_____
_____
_____

Day: _____   Date: __/__/___

1. Today's message to myself:
_____

2. Someone I could surprise with a note, gift or sign of appreciation and why:
_____

3. Today I am grateful for:
_____
_____
_____
_____

Day: _____   Date: __/__/___

1. Today's message to myself:
_____

2. Someone I could surprise with a note, gift or sign of appreciation and why:
_____

3. Today I am grateful for:
_____
_____
_____
_____

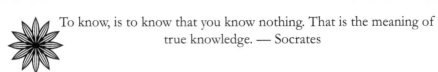

To know, is to know that you know nothing. That is the meaning of true knowledge. — Socrates

Day: _____   Date: __/__/____

1. Today's message to myself:

_____

2. Someone I could surprise with a note, gift or sign of appreciation and why:

_____

3. Today I am grateful for:

_____

_____

_____

_____

Day: _____   Date: __/__/____

1. Today's message to myself:

_____

2. Someone I could surprise with a note, gift or sign of appreciation and why:

_____

3. Today I am grateful for:

_____

_____

_____

_____

Day: _____   Date: __/__/____

1. Today's message to myself:

_____

2. Someone I could surprise with a note, gift or sign of appreciation and why:

_____

3. Today I am grateful for:

_____

_____

_____

_____

> Love does not alter the beloved, it alters itself.
> — Soren Kierkegaard

Day: _____   Date: __/__/___

1. Today's message to myself:

2. Someone I could surprise with a note, gift or sign of appreciation and why:

3. Today I am grateful for:

Day: _____   Date: __/__/___

1. Today's message to myself:

2. Someone I could surprise with a note, gift or sign of appreciation and why:

3. Today I am grateful for:

Day: _____   Date: __/__/___

1. Today's message to myself:

2. Someone I could surprise with a note, gift or sign of appreciation and why:

3. Today I am grateful for:

Printed in Great Britain
by Amazon